ALL NATURAL SOAP MAKING

ULTIMATE GUIDE TO CREATING NOURISHING NATURAL SOAP AT HOME FOR YOU AND YOUR FAMILY

PLUS 25 AMAZING SOAP RECIPES

Copyright © 2016 Laura K. Courtney

All Rights Reserved. No part of this book may be reproduced or used in any form or by any means without written permission from the author.

TABLE OF CONTENTS

Introduction	1
Safety measures for soap making	3
Common soap making terms	5
Methods of soap making	**11**
Melt and pour	11
Cold process	12
Hot process	13
Rebatching	14
Equipments	**15**
Melt and pour soap recipes	**16**
Coconut milk with Shea butter soap recipe	17
Honey and citrus soap recipe	19
Shea butter vanilla coffee soap recipe	21
Organic calendula and goat milk soap recipe (for babies)	23
Honey almond oatmeal soap recipe	25
Shaving soap recipe (for men)	27
Spicy essential oil soap recipe (for men)	30
Fruits and herbs with glycerin soap recipe	32
Cilantro soap recipe	34
Peaches and goat milk soap recipe	36
Cold process soap recipes	**38**
Goat's milk soap recipe	39
Carrot and honey soap recipe	42
Lavender colloidal oatmeal soap recipe	45

Coconut milk soap recipe 48

Buttermilk bastille soap recipe (for babies) 51

Aloe chamomile soap recipe (for babies) 53

Coffee scrub soap recipe 56

Camellia oil and coconut milk soap recipe 58

Carrot shea butter soap recipe(for babies) 61

Activated charcoal soap recipe 63

Aloe vera soap recipe 66

Spiced soap recipe (for men) 68

Citrus scotch ale soap recipe (for men) 71

Hot process soap recipes 74

Pumpkin spice soap recipe 75

Sea mud soap recipe 78

INTRODUCTION

Soap does more than getting dirt off the skin. It can also exfoliate, cleanse and heal the skin of certain skin conditions. Making your home made soap gives you the opportunity to add additional ingredients such as moisturizing agents, essential oils, herbal supplement and ingredients that exfoliate and cleanse the skin. And it will make it easy to improve the quality of your aromatherapy while bathing and to suit your own personal health needs. Commercial cheap stuff that you buy at the grocery store is anything but real soap. They are just chemicals cocktails made of disturbing synthetic ingredients that dehydrate and age the skin. While some of it causes allergic reactions, others have been linked to various forms of cancer. Therefore, all natural organic handmade soap is the real soap.

Making your own soap can be very rewarding. The good thing about soap making is that, you get to choose the ingredients and fragrances you like to use to make your own soap. And you also realize that soap making can be simple and it saves you much money, because you have to pay more if you want to buy really quality soap. Making your own soap will also allow you to add additional value to your homemade soap naturally i.e. a good proportion of glycerin and other goodies. Even the most sensitive skin can tolerate homemade soap, not to mention the fact that you can create any soap that suit your taste, by directly controlling all the ingredients and designs because only you knows what you really need.

Using homemade soap will end or reduce the skin problems that are caused by irritating chemical ingredients in commercial soap. Organic soap contains properties that would give you soothing relief from stress and tension and powerful healing to your skin. Skin conditions such as acne, psoriasis and eczema can be treated with homemade organic soap. Homemade soap will also put a stop to itchy dry skin.

Soap making can be super fun and addictive. Not to mention the fact that you can personally make soap that would rejuvenate, refresh and revitalize your skin and also give you the fresh natural scent you love so much. As you are making quality soap for yourself and your family, you can also share your homemade soap with friends. You may decide to start your own business of soap making and packaging. Selling handmade organic soap is certainly a sure way to make more money.

SAFETY MEASURES FOR SOAP MAKING

- Before you start making your soap, you need to understand the dangers of Lye (Sodium Hydroxide). Lye is an extremely corrosive and caustic chemical that is used for the Cold Process and the Hot Process soap making methods.

- Do not let the chemical touch you in any way because it will burn your skin upon contact.

- Wear protective clothing like extremely thick outwear, rubber gloves and safety goggles to avoid any contact with Lye or other harmful substances.

- Be sure to add lye to water and not water to lye, to avoid caustic eruption.

- Ensure that a bottle of vinegar is by your side. If you spill Lye, quickly pour vinegar over the mess to neutralize the chemical.

- Other soap making ingredients like essential oils can be dangerous too. Therefore, you need to understand all your ingredients and ensure you have the accurate measurement and formula.

- Make all your soap making equipments and ingredients ready in the work area before you start your soap making.

- Do not forget to label all equipments as FOR SOAP MAKING USE ONLY and store all the dangerous substances in a safe place that is far from children's reach.

- Be sure to re-run all ingredients in the Lye calculator before making your soap.

- Ensure to make your soap in an area with good ventilation because of the fumes that your Lye solution preparation is likely to produce.

- Do not inhale the fumes that would be produced when you make lye solution.

- Eliminate everything that can distract you, this includes children and pets. Educate your family members on soap making, the dangers that are involved and how to practice safety during soap making.

- Avoid cutting yourself, getting burnt with hot soap and don't leave the work area unattended.

- Be sure to measure soap ingredients by weight not volume.

COMMON SOAP MAKING TERMS

Additives

Additives are the ingredients added to soap, which are not part of soap molecules. These ingredients exclude lye, water, oils, fats and butters. Examples of additives are fragrances, colorants, preservatives, herbs, micas, salt and so on.

CP

CP stands for Cold Process soap making method which involves making soap from scratch, using Lye (Sodium Hydroxide), liquid and oils. The ingredients are separately brought to desired temperature, mixed together and allowed to saponify without additional heat.

Curing/Cure

Curing soap or to allow soap to cure is done by setting soap out in a place where air can circulate around the soap bar to enable liquid evaporation to take place on soap and for the bar to become harder. This will make the soap to become gentler on the skin and give it a better lather. Four to six weeks is the recommended cure time for Cold Process soap making.

Discount

Discount is a reduction in the amount of an ingredient. Using less water than the original amount is called Water discount. Water discounting allows a shorter curing and drying time, because there would be less water to be evaporated from the soap bar. Lye can also be discounted to allow excess oil as moisturizers. Discounts are shown in percentage.

DOS

DOS stands for Dreaded Orange Spots. It is the orange or brown color that appears as spot on soap. DOS remains a mystery as to why it occurs. While some soap makers believed that soaps made with high amounts of certain oils that include sunflower, canola and vegetable oils tend to get DOS more often than others. DOS may occur in soap that has been superfatted too much.

EO

EO (Essential Oils) is used to fragrance soap and other body products. Essential oils are considered the most natural fragrance option as they were either steam or chemically instilled from plants. They include Lavender oil, Bergamot oil, Tea Tree oil, chamomile oil, Rosemary etc.

Gel

Soaps gel during the early phase of saponification process. It becomes clear and looks like Vaseline. Not all soaps gel but milk soap generally gel no matter what you do. Other soaps might be force to gel by covering and insulation. But not to worry, soap that does not gel will still be lovely but softer when cutting, it will become hard later.

HP

HP is Hot Process method of making soap. This method involves cooking Cold Process soap to speed up saponification of the soap. This can be done in the oven (OHP) or Crockpot (CPHP). HP soaps appear rustic and they can be used as soon as they are cooled.

Lye

Lye which is also Sodium Hydroxide, NaOH and caustic soda is the base or alkaline used in making soap bars. Lye is highly corrosive and needs to be handled with care. Rubber gloves and eye protector should be used when handling lye and making soap. Lye can eat through metal and wood, therefore stainless steel, heat resistant plastic or silicone pots and tools should be used during soap making. Avoid using glass for mixing lye solution or making soap batter because heat causes weakness in glass over time.

Lye calculator

This is used to create new recipes. It calculates the amount of lye required to convert a specified amount of oils and fats to soap. Make sure you re-run all ingredients in the Lye calculator before making your soap.

Potash

Potash which is also called Potassium Hydroxide, KOH and caustic potash is the base used in making liquid soaps in place of lye used in hard soaps. Potash allows liquid soaps to stay liquid compared to Lye. The same safety precautions for working with lye should be used when working with potash.

PPO

PPO is the acronym for Per Pound of Oils. PPO is commonly used when referring to the usage rates for essential oils and fragrance.

Rancidity

Soaps that contain too much superfatted food or other organic items go rancid (spoil) in a short period of time. It can appear as DOS or mold and give a foul odor. Some delicate oils can also cause rancidity in soaps over time.

Rebatching

This is the process of melting existing soaps to create new soaps. This process is often used when soap didn't come out well or as expected. You can rebatch the soap by melting down the soap and adding additional oils to correct lye imbalance and salvaging the soap.

Saponification

Saponification is the chemical reaction that occurs between lye and fatty acids that results in formation of glycerin and soap.

Sap value

Saponification value is the milligrams of lye needed to completely saponify one gram of a specific fat. When you are making your own soap, you should know the sap value for all oils you are using in your soap, so that the oils and lye would be balance. It is also important to note that this number is different for lye (solid soap) and Potassium Hydroxide (liquid soap).

Seizing

This is a sign that something has gone wrong with your soap making. When soap seizes, it turns to thick, nearly solid state (like thick mashed potatoes) from the normal smooth, liquid consistency. This is usually caused by some fragrance oils that were added, ingredients or issues with the temperatures of the soap.

Superfatting

Superfat refers to the amount of oils remaining after saponification. Soap is superfatted by adding additional oils to it beyond what is required in order to use up all of the lye. This result in a moisturizing bar, but using too much extra oil can produce greasy and ugly soaps.

Super heaters

Super heaters are items like milk, beer, sugar and honey, that when added to soap, make it heat up quickly and also speeds trace. Be careful because adding too much super heaters may cause the soap to separate in the mold.

Swirling

Swirling is mostly used when coloring soap with color variegation, you can swirl by funnels, ITP, side by side, etc.

Trace

Trace is the point where the mixed oils and lye have combined and saponification begins. The point at which the chemical reaction has started and ingredients cannot be separated from each other. Trace can be identified when you drizzle some of the soap batter on the surface of the rest of your batch and it settles on top for a moment before it sink back into the mixture.

METHODS OF SOAP MAKING

There are many methods of making soap and this includes; Melt and Pour, Cold Process, Hot Process and Rebatching.

MELT AND POUR

Melt and Pour is the easiest and safest method of making soap. It is the process of melting a soap base that has already been made. You can add color, essential oils and fragrances as you desired with the right measurement. Mix thoroughly and pour the soap batter into molds. Once it has fully cooled and hardened, the soap can be used right away.

Start with melt and pour method of soap making if you are a beginner. The good thing about Melt and Pour method of soap making is that you don't have to handle Lye (Sodium Hydroxide), coloring and fragrances option. This method is child friendly but there should always be an adult supervision during soap making.

It is hard to mess up while making melt and pour soap because the soap base is already made. Therefore, you don't have to worry about lye calculation, recognizing trace, superfatting and other things difficult things involved with soap making.

This method would be an ideal project for kids that want to make special gift for loved ones on occasions and days such as fathers' day. A child who wants to make soap should be old enough to hold his/her container and should be supervised and helped with the melting process.

Melt and pour method of soap making also has its own disadvantage. You don't have complete control over the ingredients use in pre-made soap base you are buying. Some of these soap bases are produced with ingredients that contain chemicals that are harsh on the skin and can also cause various reactions on the skin. Therefore, you should carefully check for the ingredients used in making the melt and pour soap base you are buying and ensure you are buying the right ones.

COLD PROCESS

Cold Process soap making is a true method of making soap base because it involves creating your own soap base from scratch. It begins with mixing fixed oils like coconut oil, olive oil and palm oil with alkali (Lye or Sodium Hydroxide). First of all, the Lye solution and oil mixture must be brought to similar temperatures like 90° F. The mixture results in a chemical process called saponification. Saponification occurs when the composition of the oils and lye change to produce a soap bar. After the Lye and oils have been combined, you will blend the mixture with a whisk, stainless steel/plastic/silicone spatula or stick blender until it reaches Trace. You then pour the soap base into soap molds.

The major benefits of Cold Process method of making soap is that, you have complete control over the ingredients you will use. You get to choose the right oils, vitamins, herbs, additives and fragrances that are great for any skin type. The Cold Process method of making soap results in a long lasting soap bar, depending on the ingredients used. This method also ensures that natural ingredients are better preserved.

Using this method of soap making will give you soap bars that are creamier and luxurious because you have the freedom to research the ingredients and experiment till you get your desired soap. You can also create bars that can heal specific skin problems such as acne, dry or oily skin and other skin ailments with this method.

Cold process soap making allows different levels of artistry which include decorating soaps with swirls, making layers of colors and making all sorts of interesting designs and shapes. This method of soap making is undoubtedly the best method for producing high quality soaps.

Serious safety precautions must be taken when using the chemicals such as Lye and not all essential oils, fragrances and colorants survive in Cold Process. The use of a heating element to melt oil and thermometer to check temperatures are required. This process involves 4 to 6 weeks of curing time before the soap can be used.

HOT PROCESS

This method of soap making speeds up the time it takes for the soaps to become hard. However, this method is similar to the Cold Process. When using this method, heat is applied at different stages of soap making with the use of crockpot, oven or microwave. You begin this method with melting the oils and blending with Lye solution in a crockpot. When the soap reaches trace, you will turn on the heat and let it cook on low for 45 – 60 minutes. When soap batter becomes thick and kind of translucent, you will then scoop your soap batter into soap mold and allow it to cool. Note that more time is needed when you are using this method because you will have to watch over the soap and stir frequently while cooking it. Hot process soap doesn't take a long time to cure like cold process soap. It can be used in few days from the time it was made. Some soap makers believed that soaps made with hot process method can be used immediately it becomes firm.

The downfall of this method is that you won't create a pretty soap because the soap might appear a bit rustic and not as smooth as the cold Process method and most soap design ideas are not possible with this method of soap making. Also, some vital nutrients in some of the soap ingredients might be lost while cooking the soap.

REBATCHING

This method is also known as the hand milling method. It is the act of processing the batch of soap you previously made. It involves grating up the soap, melting it, adding more ingredients and remolding it. This technique allows the addition of delicate additives and other ingredients that could obviously be destroyed during Cold Process soap making.

This method of soap making is also used to save batches that are unsuccessful or ruined in one way or the other, for instance, you forgot to add a particular oil or fragrance to your batch. However, rebatching is best done when soap is still fresh, otherwise you will need to add liquid to the soap if it's more than seven days old.

EQUIPMENTS

- Rubber gloves
- Safety goggles
- Thick outer wear
- Accurate digital scale
- Crockpot (hot process method)
- Stainless steel pot / heat resistant plastic container (lye solution)
- Stainless steel pot (melting oils or soap blocks)
- Large stainless steel / plastic / silicone spoon(lye solution)
- Thermometer
- Stainless steel spoons (measurement)
- Small beakers / measuring cups
- Plastic bowls for (measuring oils)
- Small whisks / spoons
- Large stainless steel / plastic ladle
- Soap mold(s)
- Stick blender
- Paper / old towels
- Microwave / burner
- Knife / soap cutter
- Vinegar

MELT AND POUR SOAP RECIPES

- Coconut milk with Shea butter recipe
- Honey and citrus soap recipe
- Shea butter vanilla coffee soap recipe
- Organic calendula and goat milk soap recipe (for babies)
- Honey almond oatmeal soap recipe
- Shaving soap recipe (for men)
- Spicy essential oil soap recipe (for men)
- Fruits and herbs with glycerin soap recipe
- Cilantro soap recipe
- Peaches and goat milk soap recipe

COCONUT MILK WITH SHEA BUTTER SOAP RECIPE

Shea butter is naturally rich in vitamins A, E and F. It is so good for the skin because it offers UV protection and provides essential fatty acids and nutrients necessary for collagen production on the skin. It also helps soothe dry skin. Coconut milk has soothing properties and is a great moisturizer for dehydrated skin. It helps in treating skin ailments such acne, eczema, psoriasis, burns, dry and irritated skin. It also contains nutrients that slow down aging process such as wrinkles, age spots and sagging skin and help to improve skin elasticity. Coconut milk with Shea butter soap recipe smells heavenly and it has a rich lather that will make your skin feel smooth and soft. This homemade recipe will give you a luxuriously rich creamy and conditioning soap bar. I will give instructions on using melt and pour method for this recipe on this page.

INGREDIENTS

- Shea butter melt & pour soap base (10 oz.)
- Coconut milk powder (2 tablespoon)
- Vitamin E (2 capsules)
- Coconut fragrance oil (10 drops)

DIRECTIONS

- Cut your Shea butter melt and pour soap base into cubes and place them in a stainless steel pot or glass measuring cup.

- Heat the soap base lightly on a burner until it has completely melted (you can also use microwave to melt). Don't let the soap boil before removing from heat. Then stir it.

- Add your coconut milk powder to the melted soap base and mix thoroughly.

- Next and coconut fragrance oil and oil of vitamin E to your soap batter and stir.

- Pour it into soap mold(s) and allow soap to sit for 1 – 2 hours.

- Unmold the soap, cut if necessary and you can start using it right away.

HONEY AND CITRUS SOAP RECIPE

This soap recipe is one of my favorites due to my love for citrus scent. It also contains ingredients such as honey soap base, lemon and orange essential oils that are beneficial to the skin. Honey has antibacterial properties that kill bacteria that may cause acne and helps to heal skin faster. It also repairs damaged skin, boosts complexion and fights aging. Lemon and orange essential oils have a wonderful refreshing scent of citrus. These essential oils are taken from plants for their healing properties. They contain antibacterial properties which help to soothe itchiness and improve acne and oily skin. They also help to relieve eczema and similar skin conditions too. The honey and citrus soap recipe will produce a soap that would make your skin smooth and radiant.

I often use melt and pour method to create this handmade soap because it is easier and you can customize it with any colorant or fragrance you want. For this recipe, use honey glycerin soap, lemon essential oil and orange essential oil.

INGREDIENTS

- Honey glycerin melt and pour soap base (20 oz.)
- Lemon essential oil (10 drops)
- Orange essential oil (10 drops)
- Yellow soap colorant (2 drops)

DIRECTIONS

- Cut your honey glycerin soap base into cubes and place them in a stainless steel pot. Melt down the soap on a burner (you can use microwave too). Stir continuously until every soap base has completely melted. Do not allow soap to boil.

- Remove from heat once all soap blocks are completely melted. Mix lemon and orange essential oils and yellow soap colorant with the melted soap.

- Pour your soap into molds and leave it for about 1 – 2 hours to sit.

- Remove from molds, cut if necessary and enjoy your gentle and nourishing soap.

SHEA BUTTER VANILLA COFFEE SOAP RECIPE

This recipe would produce a sweet smelling exfoliating and anti ageing soap bar. Shea butter vanilla coffee soap is great for a sensitive skin because coffee contains antioxidant properties which exfoliates, cleanses and moisturizes the skin. It also helps to remove smells such as fish, onions and garlic from the hand and body. Apart from the fact that it helps to soothe itchy skin, smooth heels and rough feet, it also fights ageing and keeps skin fresh and glowing.

Vanilla essential oil has great properties which includes antibacterial properties great for the treatment of acne. It is rich in antioxidants which cleanse the skin, heal damaged skin and slow down signs of aging such as wrinkles, fine lines and age spots. Vanilla essential oil is also used in treating wounds, cuts and burns. Its richness in vitamin B complex such as vitamin B6, niacin, thiamin and pantothenic acid would help you maintain a healthy and radiant skin. Vitamin E is a vital antioxidant that is excellent for protecting and healing the skin. It also promotes cell and tissue repair and provides nutrients and moisture to the body.

INGREDIENTS

- Shea butter melt and pour soap base (8.5 oz.)
- Coffee grounds (2 tablespoon)
- Vitamin E (2 capsules)
- Olive oil (1 teaspoon)
- Vanilla essential oil (2 drops)

DIRECTIONS

- Cut the Shea butter soap base into cubes and place them in a stainless steel pot. Melt the soap blocks on a burner or microwave till it's completely melted. Be sure not to boil soap. Stir the melted soap.

- Add the coffee grounds, vitamin E and olive oil into the melted soap and stir to distribute the ingredients well.

- Add vanilla essential oil or any essential oil you like into the mixture and stir thoroughly.

- Pour the mixture into the soap molds and leave it to sit for about 1 – 2 hour.

- When soap becomes firm, remove from molds and your wonderful smelling soap is ready to be used.

ORGANIC CALENDULA AND GOAT MILK SOAP RECIPE (FOR BABIES)

Most baby soaps in the market are full of chemicals and synthetic petroleum based ingredients. You can actually get all natural baby soap with organic ingredients on market, but they are extremely costly. It is advisable to make your own organic baby soap. Organic calendula extract has anti bacterial properties which help to relief nappy rash on babies. It is also great for sensitive skin and on baby's skin because it moisturizes and softens the skin.

All natural Hydrolyzed oats help to hydrate the skin. It has powerful properties that naturally moisturizes the skin and reduces wrinkles and fine lines. On the other hand, goat milk also moisturizes and soothes dry and damaged skin. It is loaded with essential nutrients and vitamins such as vitamin C, D, E, B6 and B 12 that are good for the skin. Therefore, calendula and goat milk soap recipe is a lovely soap for babies, toddlers and even adults with sensitive skin.

INGREDIENTS

- Goat milk melt and pour soap base (11 oz.)
- Hydrolyzed oats (1 tablespoon)
- Olive oil (1 teaspoon)
- Organic calendula extract (1 teaspoon)

DIRECTIONS

- Cut your goat milk melt and pour soap base into cubes.

- Place it in a microwave jug and melt it in the microwave for 30 seconds, Remove from microwave and stir it. Microwave it for another 10 seconds and stir again. Repeat the process until soap blocks are completely melted. Be careful not to boil soap. You can also place your soap base cubes in a stainless steel pot and melt on the burner with low to medium heat.

- Once the soap base is melted, add the olive oil, hydrolyzed oats and calendula extract.

- Stir the mixture until all ingredients are well combined.

- Pour the mixture into mold(s).

- Spray with alcohol to remove bubbles on the surface of the mixture (no need to do this, if you don't like it).

- Leave it in a safe place to sit for 24 hours or more.

- Remove from mold(s) and let your baby enjoy your soap.

HONEY ALMOND OATMEAL SOAP RECIPE

Oatmeal has great properties that are great for the skin. They soothe the skin, reduce inflammation and heal itchy dry skin. They also help to improve skin conditions such as eczema, acne and psoriasis. Honey has great benefits for all skin type because it helps the skin to retain moisture and elasticity and is perfect for dry skin. While sweet almond oil is great for a sensitive skin and help to protect the skin and keep it soft and supple. Sweet almond oil also contains vitamin A that help to heal acne, eczema, psoriasis, skin rashes and other similar skin conditions. Honey almond oatmeal soap is great for skin care and will make your skin look smooth and flawless. I would describe using melt and pour method for this recipe.

INGREDIENTS

- Shea butter melt and pour soap base (10 oz.)
- Oatmeal (3 tablespoon)
- Honey (2 tablespoon)
- Rice bran oil (½ tablespoon)
- Sweet almond fragrance (5 drops)
- Vitamin E (2 capsules)

DIRECTIONS

- Cut the goat milk soap base into cubes.

- Place in a stainless steel pot and melt on a burner or microwave till it completely melted. Then stir.

- Add your oatmeal into the melted soap and stir to distribute evenly.

- Add sweet almond fragrance, honey, rice bran oil and vitamin E oil into the mixture.

- Mix thoroughly to distribute the ingredients.

- Pour the mixture into soap molds and allow soap to become firm for 1 – 2 hours.

- When it becomes firm, remove from molds and you can start using your soap immediately.

SHAVING SOAP RECIPE (FOR MEN)

This recipe produces an off white, creamy color with flecks of golden brown from oatmeal. It has a clean fresh manly smell. After I experimented with this recipe and produced a shaving soap for my husband, he had stop using commercial shaving cream since then. He had less irritations and no cut from using the soap. It is soothing and moisturizing to his skin. I used melt and pour method for this recipe.

The blends of lemongrass, clove and sage essential oils will make a light and clean scent that doesn't linger for too long but will be very soothing to smell while shaving. Vitamin E is a vital antioxidant that is excellent for protecting and healing the skin. It also promotes cell and tissue repair and provides nutrients and moisture to the body. Hemp seed oil is a powerful natural healer that has the perfect blends of essential fatty acids that is needed by the skin. It also has anti-inflammatory properties which makes it good for a shaving soap. Shea butter moisturizes and protects the skin. While sage essential oil has a fresh scent, it also has anti-inflammatory properties and is soothing to the skin and also contains anti- bacterial properties too. Lemongrass essential oil contains a natural antiseptic property and a pleasing fragrance. Oatmeal has exfoliating and soothing properties which help skin irritation and itching. A combination of these ingredients will produce an excellent manly shaving soap.

INGREDIENTS

- White melt and pour soap base (16 oz.)
- Finely ground whole oats (¼ cup)

- Vitamin E (3 capsules)
- Hemp seed oil (1 teaspoon)
- Olive oil (1 teaspoon)
- Lemongrass essential oil (15 drops)
- Sage essential oil (15 drops)
- Clove essential oil (10 drops)

DIRECTIONS

- Cut your white melt and pour soap base into cubes.

- Place it into a stainless steel pot and melt on a burner on medium heat. You can also use a micro wave to melt the soap base. Do not boil the soap because soap that is too hot tends to burn off essential oils and reduce the soap quality.

- Once the soap base cubes are completely melted, pour your finely ground oatmeal into the melted soap and stir till the powder disperses through the mixture.

- Add your olive oil, hemp seed oil and vitamin E oil into the mixture and stir again.

- Add required drops of lemongrass, clove and sage essential oils and mix thoroughly.

- Pour soap into molds.

- Allow soap to sit for an hour or two.

- Unmold your soap, cut if necessary and enjoy.

SPICY ESSENTIAL OIL SOAP RECIPE (FOR MEN)

If you want a medicinal spicy soap with masculine aroma for your man, try out this soap recipe. It contains cedar wood, bay, orange and lime essential oils. Cedar wood essential oil has high aromatic qualities. It helps to improve skin conditions like acne and eczema. It's antiseptic and inflammatory properties help to protect the skin against bacterial and make it possible to be used in treating wounds. Bay essential oil is medicinal spicy oil which is a good skin toner. Its anti inflammatory qualities help to relief pain and keep the body warm. Orange and cinnamon essential oils help to nourish dry and acne prone skin. Orange essential oil also promotes feeling of happiness and warmth. It is used in aromatherapy to help soothe tensed muscles and lift depression.

INGREDIENTS

- Shea butter melt and pour soap base (40 oz.)
- Cedar wood essential oil (¼ teaspoon)
- Bay essential oil (¼ teaspoon)
- Orange essential oil (¼ teaspoon)
- Cinnamon essential oil (¼ teaspoon)
- Clove essential oil (10 drops)
- Rubbing alcohol (optional)

DIRECTIONS

- Cut your Shea butter melt and pour soap base into a glass of measuring cup and microwave for 30 seconds. Stir it and microwave for another 10 seconds. Stir again and repeat the process until the soap cubes are completely melted. You can also place the cubes of the soap base in a stainless steel pot and melt on a burner.

- Stir the melted soap base and be sure not to boil the soap base.

- Add essential oils and stir.

- Pour the mixture into molds.

- Then spray lightly with rubbing alcohol to remove bubbles on the surface of the soap batter (this is optional).

- Leave your soap in a safe place to harden for an hour or two.

- Remove soap from molds and you can start using your soap immediately.

FRUITS AND HERBS WITH GLYCERIN SOAP RECIPE

Glycerin soap is one of the most moisturizing soaps. It great for all skin types and can be used by the most sensitive skin. Using glycerin soap on a regular basis will help to heal skin problems like eczema and psoriasis, and make your skin become softer and suppler. Cinnamon and lime essential oils are rich in antioxidants that help to reduce free radical damage and slow down aging process. They also help to detoxify the skin and soothe rashes, irritations and allergic reactions on skin.

Fruits such as lemon and orange protect skin from harmful sun rays and free radicals. They help to heal skin problems such as acne, dry and oily skin. Citrus helps to naturally whiten the skin and can lighten dark spots and blemishes on skin. They also have anti aging qualities. Herbs such as rosemary and basil help to combat premature aging by increasing skin elasticity. They help to protect skin cells from damage caused by free radicals and sun rays, and also great for soothing acne and other skin problems.

Therefore, fruits and herbs with glycerin soap will help rejuvenate your skin, making it a healthy and glowing skin.

INGREDIENTS

- Glycerin soap base (10 oz.)
- Herbs and fruits such as rosemary, basil, mint, orange and lemon
- Lime essential oil (15 drops)
- Cinnamon essential oil (15 drops)

DIRECTIONS

- Wash the herbs and fruits.

- Puree separately in a food processor. Add 1 – 2 tablespoons of water to the herbs while making puree. Squeeze out excess water and set it aside.

- Cut your glycerin soap base into cubes and place them in a stainless steel pot. Melt on a burner on medium heat so as not to boil soap (you can also use microwave to melt the soap blocks).

- When the soap base is completely melted, add in the fruits and herbs purees and mix until the purees is distributed.

- Add lime and cinnamon essential oil and mix thoroughly.

- Pour the mixture into molds and let it sit for an hour or two.

- Unmold soap and you can start using your homemade soap right away.

CILANTRO SOAP RECIPE

Cilantro has a pleasant aroma. It's antiseptic, antifungal, antioxidant and detoxifying properties help to clear skin disorder such as, dryness, eczema and fungal infection. Lime essential oil help to revitalize and protects skin from infection with its antioxidant and antibiotic properties. It also helps skin conditions such as acne and blemishes and reduces dark spot on the skin. Lime essential oil work as a toner for oily skin and has strong anti aging properties. Shea butter soap is a great moisturizer and contains nutrients necessary for collagen production for the skin. Cilantro soap smells divine and fabulous and will give you a glowing complexion.

INGREDIENTS

- Shea butter melt and pour soap base (16 oz.)
- Fresh chopped cilantro (3 tablespoon)
- Vitamin E (2 capsules)
- Lime essential oil (20 drops)

DIRECTIONS

- Cut your Shea butter soap base into cubes.

- Place them in a stainless steel pot and melt on a burner on medium heat. You can also use microwave to melt. Don't let the soap boil before you remove it from the heat.

- Add your fresh cilantro, lime essential oil and vitamin E into the melted soap and stir to disperse the ingredients.

- Pour the mixture into soap molds and leave it for an hour or two to become firm.

- Remove from molds and your soap is ready to be used.

PEACHES AND GOAT MILK SOAP RECIPE

Goat milk soap contains vitamin A and AHA which boast anti-aging properties on skin and is great for keeping skin moisturized and healthy. Goat milk soap is also gentle and mild for all skin type and usually safe for people with sensitive skin and skin conditions like eczema or psoriasis. Peach fragrance oil is heavenly and it has anti aging properties too. It contains vitamin A and C which help skin to retain moisture and maintain elasticity. Peach fragrance oil heals dry skin and is great for sensitive skin. The soap recipe will produce fresh scented soaps which will make your skin look radiant and healthy.

INGREDIENTS

- Goat milk melt and pour soap base (10 oz.)
- Peach soap colorant (2 drops)
- Vitamin E (2 capsules)
- Peach fragrance oil (10 drops)
- Rubbing alcohol (optional)

DIRECTIONS

- Cut the goat milk melt and pour soap base into cubes.

- Melt on burner or microwave.

- Add peach fragrance oil and vitamin E and stir the mixture well.

- Divide the melted soap between two measuring cups. Add peach soap colorant to one cup and mix.

- Make layered soap by pouring some soap with peach colorant into mold halfway. Once soap is cool and partially firm, add soap batter without peach colorant to the soap in the mold to create a white layer.

- Make swirl soap; when pouring the soap into mold, alternate filing the mold with small amounts of each color. Once the molds are filled, use a toothpick to swirl the colors together.

- You can spray once or twice with rubbing alcohol to remove bubbles from top of soap but this is optional.

- Keep the soap in a safe place and allow soap to become firm for one or two hours.

- Unmold soap and enjoy the sweet peach scent.

COLD PROCESS SOAP RECIPES

- Goat's milk soap recipe
- Carrot and honey soap recipe
- Lavender colloidal oatmeal soap recipe
- Coconut milk soap recipe
- Buttermilk Bastille soap recipe (for babies)
- Aloe chamomile soap recipe (for babies)
- Coffee scrub soap recipe
- Camellia oil and coconut milk soap recipe
- Carrot Shea butter soap recipe (for babies)
- Activated charcoal soap recipe
- Aloe Vera soap recipe
- Spice soap recipe (for men)
- Citrus scotch ale soap recipe (for men)

GOAT'S MILK SOAP RECIPE

Goat's milk help to reduce skin inflammation, soothe dry and damaged skin. It contains essential nutrients and vitamins that are so good for the skin. Goat's milk is great for treating acne and other skin problems such as eczema, skin patches, psoriasis, bumps, rashes etc. and it produces great soap lather. While coconut oil contains vitamin E that keep skin healthy and smooth. Its antioxidant qualities help to prevent premature aging and wrinkling of the skin. Olive oil helps to slow down aging process. It also helps to moisturize the skin and improves skin health. Geranium essential oil helps to soothe oily skin, acne eczema, dermatitis and other skin conditions. It also helps to brighten and revitalize dull skin.

If you want the soap with a nice creamy looking appearance, try making goat milk soap recipe. Homemade goat's milk soaps are really luxurious soap and will leave your skin smooth and radiant but making it is a bit difficult and sometimes results in darker color.

INGREDIENTS

- Lye (6 oz.)
- Goat's milk (13 oz.)
- Coconut oil (12 oz.)
- Olive oil (15 oz.)
- Vegetable oil (13 oz.)
- Geranium essential oil (1 oz.)

DIRECTIONS

- First of all, you need to freeze your goat's milk a day before you make your soap. You can put it in a zip-lock bag and freeze it.

- Get a stainless steel or heat resistant plastic bowl. Put this bowl in the sink or a larger bowl. Fill the sink or larger bowl with cold water and ice, then put the frozen chunks of milk in the inside bowl.

- Add lye very slowly and squish it into the milk carefully. Ensure to use a stainless steel potato masher for this step.

- Stir the mixture and keep replacing the ice in the outer bowl or sink if it melts, so that the milk will stay very cold. Don't worry if the milk turn orange or even tan to light brown, but if it turns dark brown, you may have to start over. Therefore, the milk needs to be kept cold to prevent it from scorching. Also, if you noticed an ammonia-like smell, don't worry as the smell will fade over time while soap is curing.

- Keep the lye / milk mixture on ice while you get your oils ready. Measure your oil with an accurate scale, and melt on a burner. When all oils are completely melted, leave it to cool.

- When oils and lye are cool to about 90°, slowly pour the lye and milk mixture into the oils. Mix it manually for the first 5 minutes, and then use a stick blender to mix it until you reach a light trace.

- When your soap has successfully come to a light trace, add geranium essential oil and mix.

- Pour the mixture into molds. Acrylic molds are recommended for goat's milk soap recipe as wood insulate very well.

- After about 24hours or more (depending on the sizes of your molds), you will remove your soap from molds and cut as desired (if necessary).

- Expose all sides to air for about 4 – 6 weeks to enable evaporation of excess liquids from soap. This also allows the finished product to become a hard, long lasting bar with a great lather.

CARROT AND HONEY SOAP RECIPE

Homemade carrot and honey soap has a powerful anti-aging and hydrating properties. It can be used as a gentle facial cleanser and can also be used as a body bar. Carrots contain vitamin A and antioxidant which protect the skin against various skin problems. Presence of vitamin C in carrots aids collagen production. Collagen helps to retain skin elasticity and slow down aging process. While carrot seed oil also nourishes, tightens and rejuvenates the skin.

Almond oil is great for sensitive skin and it contains vitamin E and A. The vitamins help to reduce acne, eczema, skin rash, psoriasis etc. Almond oil also help to slow down aging on skin and keep the skin soft and supple.

Honey is a natural moisturizer. It is great for acne and dry skin treatment and also helps to repair damaged skin. Its antibacterial properties help to heal acne, work as anti aging and complexion boost. A combination of these ingredients in your soap will make your skin radiant and feel silky to touch.

INGREDIENTS

- Lye (4 oz.)
- Pureed carrot (3.5 oz.)
- Water {used to cook carrot (7 oz.)}
- Pure honey (½ tablespoon)
- Coconut oil (10 oz.)
- Olive oil (13.5 oz.)
- Palm oil (3 oz.)

- Almond oil (3 oz.)
- Carrot seed essential oil (10 drops)

DIRECTIONS

- Boil carrots until they become soft. Remove from heat, then puree with a fork.

- Make a mixture of the pureed carrots and 200 ml of the cooking water in a separate container. Allow it to cool.

- Slowly add lye into the carrot puree mixture while you stir with a plastic or stainless steel spoon. Stir steadily and carefully until the lye is well combined with the carrot puree. Set the mixture aside to cool or you can place it in zinc filled with ice to aid it cooling.

- Measure out your oils except essential oil into a stainless steel pot. Melt down all oils to a liquid form on a burner with low temperature to prevent the oil from getting burnt. Allow your oils to cool down.

- When the lye/carrot puree mixture and oils are about the same temperature (80 – 90 degrees), slowly add lye mixture to the oils and stir with a stick blender.

- Stir until you bring the soap to light trace, and then add honey and carrot seed essential oil into the soap batter. Continue to stir the mixture until you reach a thick trace.

- Pour your soap batter into molds and allow hardening for 24 hours or more.

- When soaps become firm, unmold and cut as desired.

- Leave soaps in an open and safe place to cure for 4 – 6 weeks before using.

LAVENDER COLLOIDAL OATMEAL SOAP RECIPE

On this page, I will describe how you can make lavender colloidal oatmeal soap recipe with all natural oat milk. Lavender is a medicinal plant which has a powerful aroma that relaxes the body into a state of well-being. This extremely flavored aromatic herb is what the Romans use in their daily bathing rituals. Lavender's antiseptic and anti inflammatory properties help to get rid of acne, eczema, psoriasis and other similar skin problems. It helps to detoxify skin, heal burns and wounds, retain and restore skin complexion and slows down aging process. Lavender essential oil is the most used essential oil in the world.

Colloidal oatmeal is finely ground whole oats. It highly beneficial to the skin and is regarded as a natural healer. It helps to hydrate dry skin and protects skin from damage caused by free radicals. Skin conditions such as acne, psoriasis, eczema, insect bites, sunburn and even diaper rashes can be eased using colloidal oatmeal. It also has anti aging properties. Rice bran oil contains vitamin E and fatty acids which help to nourish skin, making it soft and velvety. It also hydrates the skin and improves skin elasticity.

Lavender with all natural oat milk and colloidal oatmeal soap recipe will help to nourish and rejuvenate your skin, thus giving you a radiant and youthful look.

INGREDIENTS

- Lye (4 oz.)
- Oat milk (10 oz.)

- Colloidal Oatmeal (2 tablespoon)
- Lavender buds (1 oz.)
- Coconut oil (5 oz.)
- Olive oil (10.5 oz.)
- Palm oil (5 oz.)
- Castor oil (1 oz.)
- Rice bran oil (2.5 oz.)
- Mango butter (2 oz.)
- Vitamin E (2 capsules)
- Lavender essential oil (1 oz.)

DIRECTIONS

- First, you will create your all natural oat milk; measure ½ cup of whole oat and 1½ cup of water into a container. Blend the mixture with a blender till it become a smooth white creamy liquid. Make sure you use the old fashioned whole oat and not quick oats.

- Filter the liquid with a cheese cloth or fine strainer to remove all the oat particles.

- Carefully pour your lye into the Oat milk. There would be a reaction between the two components which will cause the solution to heat up. Therefore, prepare your lye solution in the absence of children and pets, and in a well ventilated area. Stir the mixture and set it aside to cool down.

- Measure out your oils and mango butter into a stainless steel soap making pot. Melt down all oils and butter to a liquid form on a burner with low temperature of below 100 degrees F to prevent the oil from getting burnt. Allow your oils to cool down before adding them to the batch.

- Next, measure 2 tablespoons of colloidal oatmeal. You can purchase it or create your own by grinding up some whole oats into fine powder in a coffee blender.

- Pour your oat milk/lye solution into your soap making oils slowly and carefully, while stirring with a silicone or stainless steel spatula. Continue to stir it until the batch gets an even color and texture. After that, you can start mixing with a stick blender. Mix the batch until you reach a thin trace.

- Add your measured lavender essential oil and vitamin E and mix the batch again.

- Pour your colloidal oatmeal into the batch and mix thoroughly with a stick blender or you can mix manually.

- Pour the batch into acrylic mold(s). You can sprinkle some lavender buds on the top of your soap to make an adorable finished product.

- After 24 hrs, remove the soap from molds, cut if necessary and allow them to cure for about 4 to 6 week. Ensure to expose all sides of the soap to air.

COCONUT MILK SOAP RECIPE

Coconut milk has soothing properties and is a great moisturizer for dehydrated skin. It helps in treating skin ailments such acne, eczema, psoriasis, burns, dry and irritated skin. It also contains nutrients that slow down aging process such as wrinkles, age spots and sagging skin and help to improve skin elasticity. Tallow is rich in antioxidants, vitamins A, D and E that helps to nourish the skin. It's so good for the skin, as it helps to promote skin cell regeneration and delays aging process.

Calendula on the other hand helps to soothe and soften the skin. Its anti-inflammatory and anti-bacterial qualities help to soothe skin conditions such as eczema, acne, dermatitis and psoriasis. It also helps to speed up healing of wounds and minor cuts. These ingredients have similar properties and the soap recipe would give you a luxuriously rich, creamy and conditioning soap bar suitable for a sensitive and delicate skin.

INGREDIENTS

- Lye (4 oz.)
- Coconut milk (3 oz.)
- Distilled water (7 oz.)
- Tallow (5 oz.)
- Coconut oil (6 oz.)
- Olive oil (13 oz.)
- Castor oil (3 oz.)
- Palm oil (5 oz.)
- Vitamin E (2 capsules)
- Calendula flower petal (1 tablespoon)

DIRECTIONS

- Warm your coconut milk lightly and put it aside. Also grind your calendula flower petal and set it aside.

- Start by weighing your water and pouring it into a container. Then, measure the lye and slowly pour it into the water and stir continuously until the lye beads have completely dissolved.

- Measure your oils and tallow into a stainless steel pot. Melt down to a liquid form with a low temperature on the burner. Allow your melted tallow and oils to cool down to about 90° F.

- Pour the lye solution into the pots of oil slowly and carefully while stirring the mixture with a plastic or stainless steel spatula. Keep stirring in a steady motion. You can stir with a stick blender to make it faster.

- When your soap batter has reached a light trace, add your coconut milk and vitamin E oil and keep stirring.

- When your soap batter has reach medium trace, add the finely ground calendula petals into the soap and mix thoroughly.

- Pour the soap into your soap molds and leave it to sit for 24 hours or more.

- Remove from molds after 24 hours and cut if necessary. Keep your soap in a cool dry place for 4 – 6 weeks to cure before use.

BUTTERMILK BASTILLE SOAP RECIPE (FOR BABIES)

This soap recipe is great for baby's skin and people with sensitive skin. The ingredients include buttermilk which contains lactic acid that helps to soften, brighten and gently exfoliate the skin. It moisturizes the skin and help to stimulate natural collagen production on the skin.

You can also add zinc oxide which is great for itchy and irritated skin. Zinc oxide acts as sunscreen that protects the skin and keeps UV rays from penetrating the skin and causing cell damage. Its antibacterial qualities makes it effective in treating skin problems such as acne, blemishes, eczema, psoriasis and even diaper rashes. Zinc also slows down aging process by reducing wrinkles and fine lines.

Buttermilk Bastille baby soap recipe would give you a baby bar that will gently cleanse your baby's delicate skin and leaves your baby's skin clean, super soft and silky smooth.

INGREDIENTS

- Lye (2 oz.)
- Buttermilk (1 tablespoon)
- Zinc oxide (1 tablespoon)
- Distilled water (4 oz.)
- Coconut oil (4 oz.)
- Olive oil (13 oz.)
- Castor oil (3 oz.)

Note that essential oils and fragrances cannot be added into baby soap. And you can substitute any milk of your choice such as goat's milk, coconut milk and almond milk for buttermilk.

DIRECTIONS

- Make lye solution by slowly pouring your measured lye in a container of measured water. Stir until lye beads and crystals dissolve. Then, keep it aside to cool down.

- Measure the coconut oil into a stainless steel pot and place the pot on a burner to melt down the oil. Add olive oil and castor into the coconut oil when it's melted.

- Add your buttermilk powder and zinc oxide into the oils and stir to get rid of lumps.

- When the oils and lye solution cool down to below 100°, pour the lye solution into the oils. Mix with a stick blender till it reaches trace.

- Pour into molds and allow your soap to sit for about 24 hours or more.

- After 24 hours, remove your soap from mold, cut as you desired and set it in a well ventilated area to cure for about 4 – 6 weeks before using.

ALOE CHAMOMILE SOAP RECIPE (FOR BABIES)

Aloe Vera herb contains amino acids, minerals, enzymes, vitamins and other components that are great for skin care. It works as a great medicine for various skin ailments like dryness and burns. It powerful moisturizing properties will make your skin look and feel younger and suppler.

Cocoa butter soap is a great moisturizer and contains nutrients necessary for collagen production for the skin. Chamomile herb is a natural cleanser that has healing properties. It helps to soothe skin irritations, fight against acne and other skin problem and protects the skin from free radical damage. It is also a great moisturizer that helps to hydrate dry skin and promotes a healthy and radiant skin.

Rice bran oil contains vitamin E and fatty acids that helps to nourish the skin, making it soft and velvety. It is a natural moisturizer and it can be used to treat acne, eczema and other similar skin conditions. Rice bran oil also aids collagen production on the skin and protects the skin against age-related wrinkles, fine lines and dark spot. Aloe vera chamomile soap recipe would produce a soap bar that is good for babies and adults.

INGREDIENTS

- Lye (3 oz.)
- Aloe Vera gel / distilled water (8 oz.)
- Cocoa butter (6 oz.)
- Chamomile infused olive oil / olive oil (7.5 oz.)

- Palm oil (3 oz.)
- Rice bran oil (2 oz.)
- Castor oil (2 oz.)

DIRECTIONS

- First thing to do is to create a chamomile infused olive oil. Measure olive oil and chamomile flowers into a crock pot. Stir and set the crock pot to LOW. Cover the crock pot and let the chamomile flowers and olive oil cook for 30 minutes. You may infuse them a little longer in order to get all the benefits from the herbs or strain the oil from the flowers after 30 minutes.

- After infusing the oils, allow to cool slightly and then, pour through a strainer into a heat resistant bowl. Set the oil aside.

- Make lye solution by pouring the amount of lye needed into measured aloe vera gel or distilled water and mix thoroughly. Allow the mixture to cool.

- Place all your oils and cocoa butter into a stainless steel pot and heat them on a medium heat. Use a thermometer to monitor it and be sure that the temperature doesn't go over 150° F.

- Once the oils and butter is melted, remove from heat and leave to cool.

- You may monitor your lye solution with a candy thermometer. When lye solution and melted oils are about the same temperature (around 90° to 100°), pour the lye solution into the melted oils and mix with a plastic or stainless steel spatula. After few minutes, you can change it to a stick blender.

- Continue mixing until the mixture reaches a trace.

- Pour the mixture into molds and allow your soap to sit for 24 hours or more.

- Unmold soaps and cut if necessary.

- Place the soap bars on a rack to cure for 4 – 6 weeks before using.

COFFEE SCRUB SOAP RECIPE

This homemade soap is mild, soft and invigorating. It contains coffee grounds which help to exfoliate the skin by removing dead skin cells and leaving your skin smooth. Coffee ground is rich in antioxidant which helps to heal the skin of damage caused by UV rays from exposure to the sun. As much as it helps to tighten the skin and slow down aging process, it also helps to brighten skin complexion.

The vitamin E content in soybean oil helps to reduce acne scarring, appearance of blemishes and also protect the skin against sunburn. It is a great moisturizer that can improve the overall tone of the skin and helps to delay aging process. Coffee scrub soap will help to keep your skin smooth and healthy.

INGREDIENTS

- Lye (2 oz.)
- Distilled water (6 oz.)
- Coffee grounds (5 oz.)
- Coconut oil (5 oz.)
- Olive oil (5 oz.)
- Soybean oil (6 oz.)
- Vitamin E (2 capsules)
- Rosemary essential oil (¼ teaspoon)

DIRECTIONS

- Start by mixing coffee grounds in water to make coffee.

- Slowly pour your lye into the coffee and mix until the lye beads dissolves. Set it aside to cool.

- Measure your coconut oil into a stainless steel pot and heat to melt it into liquid form. Then add olive and soybean oil into the melted coconut oil.

- When the oils have cooled down, pour your lye / coffee solution into the oils and mix manually or use a stick blender. Keep mixing until the soap batter reaches a light trace.

- Add vitamin E oil and rosemary essential oil to the soap batter and mix till soap reaches a thick trace.

- Pour batter into molds and allow your soap to sit for about 24 hours or more (depending on the sizes of your molds) to saponify.

- Unmold your soap, cut if necessary and leave it in a well ventilated place for 4 – 6 weeks to cure.

CAMELLIA OIL AND COCONUT MILK SOAP RECIPE

Camellia oil has so many great properties that is great on skin and so also is coconut milk (I love the rich smell of coconut milk). This soap recipe is good for all skin types. Camellia oil is rich in vitamins A, B, D and E as well as omega 3, 6 and 9 fatty acids. It is light and absorbs quickly and thoroughly into the skin. Camellia oil works as moisturizer for dry skin, helps to soothe acne on the skin, prevents wrinkles and reduces stretch marks.

Coconut milk has soothing properties and is a great moisturizer for dehydrated skin. It helps in treating skin ailments such acne, eczema, psoriasis, burns, dry and irritated skin. It also contains nutrients that slow down aging process such as wrinkles, age spots and sagging skin and help to improve skin elasticity. Shea butter is naturally rich in vitamins A, E and F. It so good for the skin, as it offers UV protection and provides essential fatty acids and nutrients necessary for collagen production for the skin. It also helps soothe dry skin.

Homemade camellia oil and coconut milk soap is the perfect soap for a healthy, smooth and glowing skin.

INGREDIENTS

- Lye (4 oz.)
- Distilled water (7 oz.)
- Coconut milk (3.5 0z.)
- Coconut oil (6 oz.)
- Camellia oil (3 oz.)

- Olive oil (10 oz.)
- Castor oil (3 oz.)
- Palm oil (9.5 oz.)
- Vitamin E (2 capsules)
- Lemongrass essential oil (½ teaspoon)
- Tea tree essential oil (½ teaspoon)

DIRECTIONS

- Make lye solution by slowly pouring measured lye into a container that has the amount of water needed. Stir until lye beads and crystals dissolve completely. Set it aside to cool. You can place the container in the sink or larger bowl, filled it with ice water and place container of lye solution in it to speed it cooling.

- Measure your oils into a stainless steel pot or microwave bowl and melt on a low temperature to avoid burning it.

- When your oils and lye solution cool down to below 100 degrees F, pour the lye solution into the oils and stir with a stick blender or manually till it reaches a thin trace.

- Add your slightly warmed coconut milk into soap batter and continue to stir until it reaches a thin trace.

- Add essential oils and vitamin E and stir till soap reaches a thick trace.

- Pour into soap molds and allow it to sit for about 24 hours or more.

- Remove from mold, cut if necessary and place the soap bars in a well ventilated area where evaporation of liquid can take, for about 4 – 6 weeks.

CARROT SHEA BUTTER SOAP RECIPE (FOR BABIES)

Carrots contain vitamin A and antioxidant which protect the skin against various skin problems. Presence of vitamin C in carrots aids collagen production. Collagen helps to retain skin elasticity and slow down aging process. Carrots also help to nourish the skin. Shea butter is naturally rich in vitamins A, E and F. It so good for the skin as it offers UV protection and provides essential fatty acids and nutrients necessary for collagen production on the skin. It also helps soothe dry skin. Coconut and olive oils are moisturizers that help to maintain a healthy and smooth skin. Carrot soap is gentle and mild for babies and those with sensitive skin.

INGREDIENTS

- Lye (4 oz.)
- Carrot cooking / plain water (4 oz.)
- Carrots puree (4 oz.)
- Shea butter (5 oz.)
- Coconut oil (7 oz.)
- Olive oil (19 oz.)

DIRECTIONS

- Create your own carrots puree (you can simply use carrot baby food) by putting sliced carrots into a pot of water. Cover the pot and cook till carrots become tender. Spoon the carrots from water and allow cooling to room temperature. Blend the carrots with a small amount of cooking water to form puree.

- Pour carrots puree and cooking water into a stainless steel or plastic container.

- Slowing pour lye into the mixture and stir until lye beads dissolve completely.

- Measure out your oils and Shea butter in a stainless steel pot on a burner and melt the oils and butter on a low heat. Then, set it aside cool.

- Once your oils and lye / carrots puree mixture are cool to room temperature or 90 °, pour the lye solution into oils.

- Use a stick blender to stir the oils and lye solution thoroughly. Stir until soap reaches a trace.

- Pour into mold(s) and allow it to sit for 24 hour or more.

- Unmold soaps after 24 hours, cut into bars if necessary and let it cure in open air for 4 – 6 weeks.

ACTIVATED CHARCOAL SOAP RECIPE

Activated charcoal with sea salt and calcium Bentonite clay soap contains detox, cleansing ingredients and it is rich in vitamins and minerals that nourish the skin. Activated charcoal takes care of oily skin by removing toxins from the body. It is also effective in treating skin irritations such as acne and dark spots. Activated charcoal can also be used to neutralize poisonous substances ingested into the body e.g. spider or deadly snake bite. It has anti-aging properties that help to tighten pores and smooth the skin.

Activated charcoal soap is also a salt bar because it ingredients include a generous amount of Mediterranean Sea salt which is full of minerals that is beneficial to the skin. Mediterranean Sea salt helps to keep the skin moisturized and revitalized. It helps to unclog the pores and exfoliate dead skin cells. It does not only help to detoxify the body, it also helps to heal acne and other skin problems.

Calcium Bentolite clay is great for all skin types. It helps to soothe oily skin and keep the skin soft, supple and blemish free. It also unclogs the skin pores and shrinks them, giving your skin a youthful look. This clay will help to rebuild damaged skin tissue and rejuvenate skin naturally. You can make a swirl or double color soap with this recipe.

INGREDIENTS

- Lye (2.6 oz.)
- Activated charcoal (1 tablespoon)
- Calcium Bentonite clay (1 tablespoon)

- Mediterranean sea salt (8 oz.)
- Coconut milk (7 oz.)
- Coconut oil (16.5 oz.)
- Olive oil (2 oz.)
- Rice bran oil (3 oz)
- Shea butter (2.5 oz)
- Grapefruit essential oil (½ teaspoon)
- Clove essential oil (½ teaspoon)

DIRECTIONS

- Make sure your coconut milk is frozen before you start making your soap.

- Slowly add lye to the frozen coconut milk and carefully mix it.

- Measure all oils and Shea butter into a stainless steel pot and melt on a burner.

- Add the coconut milk / lye solution to the melted oils and butter.

- Use a silicone spatula or stick blender to mix the mixture until it reaches a thin trace.

- Pour your soap batter into two different containers preferably a glass measuring cup.

- Add activated charcoal in one container and Bentonite clay in the other container.

- Use a stick blender to mix well (you can mix the light color first and then the dark color to avoid washing the stick blender between mixes). Add essential oils to the Mediterranean Sea salt and mix.

- Add the Mediterranean Sea salt / essential oils to both soap batter and mix thoroughly with a spatula.

- Pour the soap batter in molds to make double color and you can add a swirl to the soap batter if you want.

- Leave your soap in a safe place to cure for 4 – 6 weeks before using.

ALOE VERA SOAP RECIPE

Aloe Vera herb contains amino acids, minerals, enzymes, vitamins and other components that are great for skin care. It works as a great medicine for various skin ailments like dryness and burns. It powerful moisturizing properties will make your skin look and feel younger and suppler. Using lard for soap making will add a creamy lather, conditioning properties and some hardness to the finished soap. Lard is an excellent moisturizer for the skin. It also contains anti-aging properties that would make your skin soft and smooth.

INGREDIENTS

- Lye (7 oz.)
- Distilled water (10 oz.)
- Aloe Vera gel purees (10 oz.)
- Coconut oil (15 oz.)
- Olive oil (13 oz.)
- Shea Butter (2.5 oz.)
- Lard (10.5 oz)
- Lavender essential oil (45 drops)
- Geranium essential oil (15 drops)

DIRECTIONS

- Get your Aloe Vera gel ready or carefully cut out the clear gel from the leaves. Add water to the gel to make puree of about 9.6 ounces.

- Make your lye solution by adding lye to water carefully and slowly. Set it aside to cool down.

- Measure olive oil, coconut oil, shea butter and lard into a stainless steel pot and melt on a burner. You can also use microwave to melt down your oils and butter. Then set it aside to cool after melting.

- When lye solution and oils have cooled to room temperature, add your lye solution to the oils and stir.

- Next add Aloe Vera gel purees to the mixture and mix thoroughly until all ingredients dispersed

- Mix the soap batter with a stick blender until it reaches a light trace.

- Add essential oils and mix till soap reaches a thick trace.

- Pour the mixture into molds and allow sitting for about 24 hours or more.

- Unmold the soaps and cut if necessary.

- Leave it on a rack to cure for about 4 – 6 weeks before using.

SPICED SOAP RECIPE (FOR MEN)

Making your own soap can be quite addictive and fun. While you make your girly scent soap, you can also make soap for the men in your life too. There are many recipes and options that will allow you to completely customize your soap to fit your needs and desires. This recipe will produce a hard moisturizing soap bar with a lot of lather. It contains tallow which has high cleansing abilities and also makes a hard bar. Tallow is rich in antioxidants, vitamins A, D and E that helps to nourish the skin. It also promotes skin cell regeneration and delays aging process.

Beeswax has many health benefits for the skin that are almost too many to count and a natural pleasing fragrance. It has anti-inflammatory properties that help to soothe, hydrate and protect skin. Its vitamins A content helps to exfoliate and rejuvenate skin. Beeswax also helps to soothe skin irritations such as acne, rosacea, eczema and other similar skin problems.

Patchouli essential oil has a strong sweet spicy and musky aroma. It can be used to treat skin problems such as dermatitis, eczema, acne and dry skin. It also helps to prevent premature aging and keep skin soft and supple. Cinnamon essential oil is rich in antioxidants that help to reduce free radical damage and slow down aging process. It also helps to detoxify the skin and soothe rashes, irritations and allergic reactions on skin. Clove essential oil is rich in minerals and vitamins A and C. It is great for acne treatment, reduces effects of aging such as wrinkles and sagging skin. It also lightens skin blemishes and rejuvenates skin.

INGREDIENTS

- Lye (4 oz.)
- Distilled water (11 oz.)
- Tallow (13 oz.)
- Beeswax (1.5 oz.)
- Coconut oil (4.5 oz.)
- Olive oil (12 oz.)
- Castor oil (4.5 oz.)
- Patchouli essential oil (0.4 oz.)
- Peppermint essential oil (22 drops)
- Clove essential oil (5 drops)

DIRECTIONS

- Pour lye into water slowly and carefully to make lye solution. Stir the mixture with a stainless steel or heat resistant plastic spatula until lye beads dissolves. Let the mixture cool to about 90 degrees. You can place it in a sink filled with ice water and monitor with a thermometer.

- Measure your ingredients except essential oils, into a stainless steel pot and heat slightly on a burner. Ensure the beeswax melt before you remove from heat. Then, let it cool.

- When the temperature of your oils and lye mixture are about the same temperature i.e. 90°, slowly pour the lye solution into the oils. Use stick blender to bring the soap batter to a light trace.

- Add essential oils and stir till it reaches a thick trace.

- Pour the mixture into your molds and leave to sit for 24 hours or more.

- Unmold your soap, cut if necessary and stand up bars in a dry area to allow circulation of air for 4 – 6 weeks curing time.

CITRUS SCOTCH ALE SOAP RECIPE (FOR MEN)

Citrus scotch ale soap recipe would give you a soap that smells more like an extremely rich caramel scent with a hint of honey and citrus. This would make perfect gifts for the men in your life. Dark beer contains vitamins and nutrients that are really good for acne reduction and helps to increase natural skin shine. It helps to remove toxins from skin and hydrates the skin. Its vitamin B content will help to smooth your skin and delay aging process.

Malted barley is rich in vitamin C, antioxidants and minerals that are extremely beneficial to the skin. It helps to preserve skin elasticity and also protect the skin against free radical damage. Barley also helps to heal skin of common skin problems and it gives the skin a pleasant tone.

Macadamia nut oil contains properties that can help to prevent wrinkles, age spots and other signs of aging. It is rich in essential fatty acids and good for all skin types as it deep cleanse the pores, moisturizes and soothe sunburn. Macadamia nut oil also offers skin protection against UV rays and free radical damage. It helps to fight acne, relieves eczema and other inflammatory skin conditions and helps to balance and control oily skin.

Grapefruit essential oil has a fresh citrus scent that is very uplifting to the body and mind. Its richness in vitamin C and antioxidants helps to neutralize free radicals that can damage the skin. It also has antiseptic qualities that help to soothe acne on skin and good for treating oily skin. Grapefruit essential oil improves blemish appearance on skin, reduces signs of aging and helps to maintain a youthful glowing skin.

INGREDIENTS

- Lye (4 oz.)
- Dark beer (9.5 0z.)
- Ground malted barley (1 tablespoon)
- Honey (1½ tablespoon)
- Coconut oil (6 oz.)
- Olive oil (10 oz.)
- Castor oil (1.5 oz.)
- Palm oil (4.5 oz.)
- Macadamia nut oil (2.5 oz.)
- Grapefruit essential oil (½ tablespoon)
- Lemon essential oil (½ tablespoon)
- Orange essential oil (½ tablespoon)
- Clove essential oil (10 drops)

DIRECTONS

- Pour your beer into a large bowl and let it sit for a day or two. If carbonation is present in the beer, it will bubble up or overflow when you mix lye with it. Therefore, it advisable to place the mixing container inside sink or a larger bowl to catch any spillage (even if you do air out your beer).

- Allow your mixture to cool down.

- Measure your oils into a stainless steel pot and melt it on a burner or microwave. Also, set it aside to cool down.

- Slowly pour your lye / beer solution into the oils and stir with a stick blender until it reach a thin trace.

- Pour your measured honey and ground malted barley into the mixture and stir till it reaches a thick trace.

- Pour the soap batter into molds and leave it in a safe place to sit for about 24 hours or more.

- After 24 hours, unmold your soaps and leave them in an open place for 4 – 6 weeks to cure before using.

HOT PROCESS SOAP RECIPES

- Pumpkin spice soap recipe
- Sea mud soap recipe

PUMPKIN SPICE SOAP RECIPE

Pumpkin is rich in fruit enzymes and alpha hydroxyl acids (AHA) which help to regenerate, brighten and smooth skin. Its antioxidant and vitamin A and C contents help to soften and soothe the skin. It also boosts collagen production to prevent the signs of aging and skin hydration. Pumpkin helps to heal acne and damages caused by free radicals and also helps to remove dark spot on skin. It exfoliates the skin and improves skin tone. Pumpkin seeds are rich in vitamin E and fatty acids which are great for good barrier function on skin.

Pumpkin pie spice is a blend of ground spices such as cinnamon, ginger, nutmeg and allspice. Cinnamon helps to reduce acne, ginger can be used to detoxify and tone skin. While nutmeg contains astringent properties that help to fight acne on skin. Allspice also has great properties that are beneficial to the skin. A combination of this ingredients will produce a bar soap that is extremely beneficial to the skin. I used hot process method for this soap recipe. Pumpkin pie spice has exfoliating properties but if you don't like exfoliating soap, you can omit the spice.

INGREDIENTS

- Lye (5 oz.)
- Distilled water (8 oz.)
- Pumpkin puree (3 oz.)
- Pumpkin pie spice (3 tablespoon)
- Coconut oil (20 oz.)
- Olive oil (10 oz.)

- Vitamin E (2 capsules)
- Tea tree essential oil (25 drops)
- Cinnamon essential oil (25 drops)

DIRECTIONS

- Start soap making by making pumpkin puree. Place a pumpkin in a pre heat oven of about 350°. Bake for one to two hours, depending on the size of your pumpkin. You will know it done when the tip of your knife stick into the skin a little. Although the skin would still be tough.

- Remove from oven and let it cool. Once it cooled (enough to handle), cut and remove seeds and stringy stuff. Scrape the skin and blend the soft flesh and seeds in your food processor or blender.

- Make lye solution. Carefully pour lye into water and stir well until lye beads dissolves. Allow it to sit for 5 – 10 minutes.

- Place coconut oil and olive oil inside a crockpot and melt oils on a low. Remove from heat and set it aside to cool.

- Carefully pour the lye solution into the melted oils and stir with a plastic or stainless steel spoon / spatula. Switch to a stick blender to bring the soap mixture to a light trace.

- Add pumpkin puree and mix till you achieved full trace.

- Turn on the heat and let it cook on low for 45 – 60 minutes. You need to stay close because it will go through bubbling, rising and frothing stages. And when it wants to boil over the top of the crockpot, stir it back down.

- After 60 minutes test soap to see if it's done. You can immerse a PH test strip and wait for few minute for it to change color. If it higher than 10, your soap is not done but if it is between 7 and10, then your soap is done. You can also pull a tiny bit of the soap out of the crock. Let it cool for a minute and touch it to your tongue. If it "zaps" you, then you need to cook it more, but if it tastes bitter and soap, it means your soap is done.

- Remove crockpot from heat. Add spices, vitamin E and essential oils and stir thoroughly.

- Scoop your soap batter into molds and allow it to sit for 24 hours or more.

- Unmold soap after 24 hours or more and into bars if necessary.

- You can use your soap immediately but waiting for a week or two to cure before using will give you a harder, long-lasting bar.

SEA MUD SOAP RECIPE

Sea mud also known as French green clay contains mineral oxides and decomposed plant materials that include seaweed and kelp. It has calcium, magnesium, potassium, phosphorous, silicon, selenium and copper. These elements work together in the soap to nourish and detoxify skin. Olive oil softens and moisturizes the skin. While coconut oil contains vitamin E that keep skin healthy and smooth. Its antioxidant qualities help to prevent premature aging and wrinkling of the skin. Ylang-ylang essential oil helps to soothe irritated skin, oily skin and acne prone skin. Sea mud soap recipe is good for all skin types and will leave you with a younger looking skin and more radiant complexion.

INGREDIENTS

- Lye (4 oz.)
- Distilled water (11 oz.)
- Sea mud (3 tablespoon)
- Coconut oil (10 oz.)
- Olive oil (20 oz.)
- Castor oil (3 oz)
- Ylang-ylang essential oil (20 drops)

DIRECTIONS

- Make lye solution by slowly adding lye to water while mixing gently. Stir until lye beads and crystals dissolves and set it aside to cool for 5 – 10 minutes.

- Measure out coconut oil and olive oil into crockpot and melt on LOW.

- Add lye solution into the crockpot and let soap cook on LOW for 45 minutes.

- Add your sea salt to the soap, mix thoroughly and cover again for some minutes.

- The soap will look a little like semi translucent Vaseline with no oil puddles in the middle when it ready.

- Test soap to see if it's done. You can immerse a PH test strip and wait for few minute for it to change color. If it higher than 10, your soap is not done but if it is between 7 and10, then your soap is done. You can also test by pulling a tiny bit of the soap out of the crockpot, let it cool for a minute and touch to your tongue. If soap taste soapy and bitter, your soap is done but if it 'zaps' you, your soap is not done and you should cook it more. It is important that you let your soap cook well for the lye to be converted. Otherwise, the finished soap can burn your skin.

- Allow soap to cool a little when it done, then add your essential oil and mix thoroughly.

- Scoop your soap into molds and allow it to cool harden for 24 hours or more. You can also keep it in the fridge to speed up this process.

- Unmold soap and cut into bars.

- Place your soap in an open dry place to cure for few days. And you can try one bar immediately.

Printed in Great Britain
by Amazon